AF256873

# Deliciously Mediterranean: A Culinary Journey through Healthy Recipes

*Discover the Flavors, Health Benefits, and Beauty of the Mediterranean Diet.*

**Elisa Cobb**

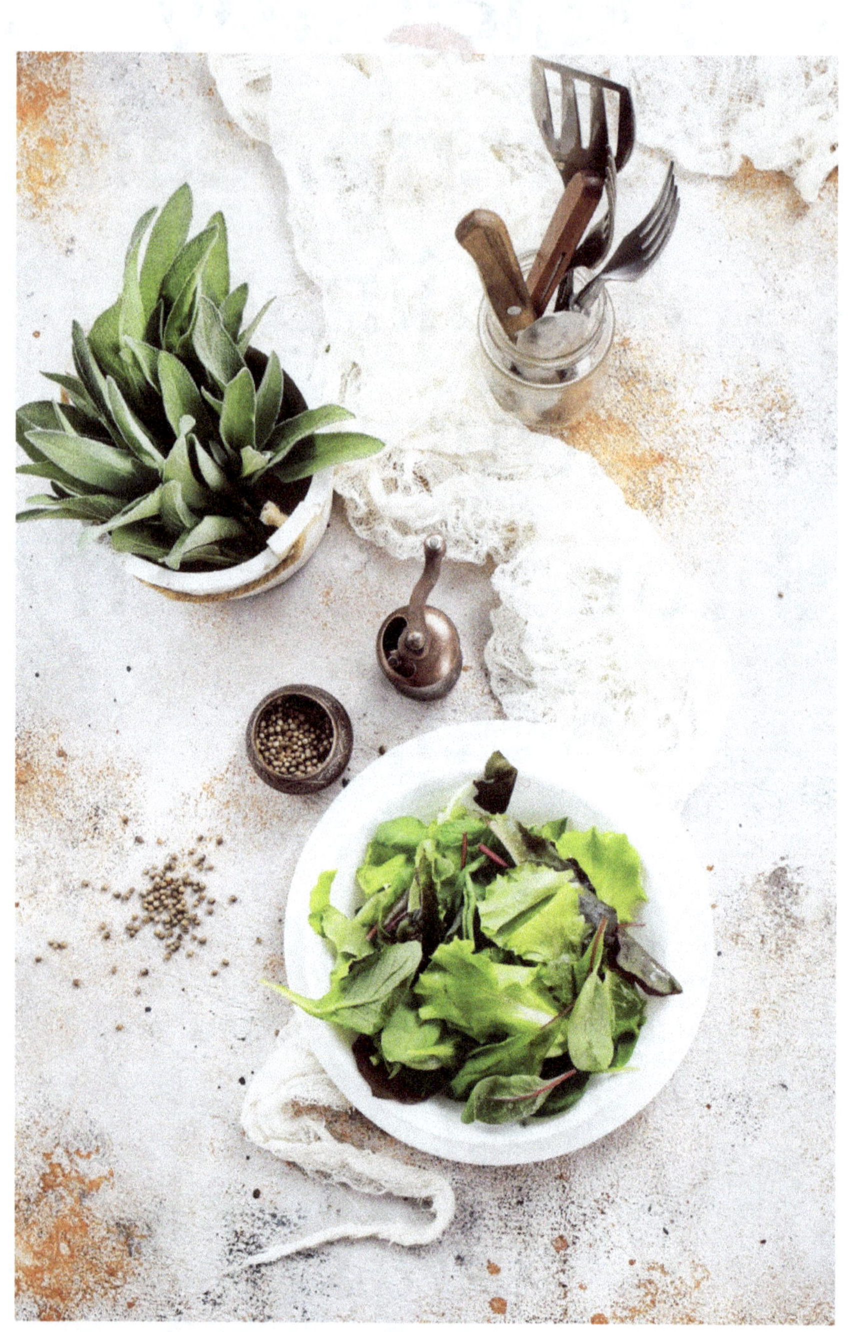

# Table of content

# MEDITERRANEAN BREAKFAST RECIPE

# Garlicky Scrambled Eggs

Total time: 25 minutes

Prep time: 10 minutes

Cooking time: 15 minutes

Yield: 2 servings

**Ingredients**

- ½ tsp. extra virgin olive oil
- ½ cup ground beef
- ½ tsp. garlic powder
- 3 eggs
- Salt
- Pepper

**Directions**

- Set a medium-sized pan over medium heat.
- Add extra virgin olive oil and heat until hot but not smoking.
- Stir in ground beef and cook for about 10 minutes or until almost done.
- Stir in garlic and sauté for about 2 minutes.
- In a large bowl, beat the eggs until almost frothy; season with salt and pepper.
- Add the egg mixture to the pan with the cooked beef and scramble until ready.
- Serve with toasted bread and olives, for a healthy, satisfying breakfast!

# Healthy Breakfast Casserole

Total time: 60 minutes

Prep time: 10 minutes

Cooking time: 50 minutes

Yield: 6 servings

**Ingredients**

- 2 tbsp. extra virgin olive oil, divided
- ½ a medium-sized onion, diced
- 2 medium-sized yellow potatoes. diced
- 1 lb. zucchini, sliced
- 3 portabella mushroom caps, diced
- 150g torn fresh spinach
- 200g ricotta
- 200g light ricotta cheese
- 2 cups of egg whites
- 12 grape tomatoes, sliced into ⅓ pieces
- 3 peeled and roasted fresh peppers, sliced
- 2 sourdough rolls
- 4 tbsp. Pecorino Romano cheese, grated
- 100g skim-milk mozzarella cheese, grated

**Directions**

- Preheat the oven to 400°F.
- Mix together olive oil, onion and potato and roast for at least 15 minutes; remove from oven and keep on the baking tray.

- In a bowl, combine together ½ tablespoon olive oil and zucchini; toss to coat well and transfer to a baking tray.
- Return all the vegetables to oven and roast for about 40 minutes or until golden in color.
- In the meantime, place ½ tablespoon olive oil in a pan and sauté mushrooms for about 4 minutes.
- Remove the cooked mushrooms from pan and set aside.
- Add the remaining olive oil to pan and sauté chopped spinach until tender.
- In a mixing bowl, combine together both types of ricotta and egg whites; set aside.
- Combine together all the vegetables, including grape tomatoes and peppers, with sourdough rolls in a 9 x 13 baking dish; top with the ricotta mixture and sprinkle with pecorino and mozzarella cheese.
- Bake for at least 40 minutes or until done. Remove from the oven, cool slightly.
- Cut into six slices and enjoy your breakfast.

# Egg and Sausage Breakfast Casserole

Total time: 1 hour, 25 minutes

Prep time: 20 minutes

Cook time: 1 hour, 5 minutes

Yield: 12 servings

**Ingredients**

**The crust:**

- 3 tbsp. olive oil, divided
- 2 lb. peeled and shredded russet potatoes
- ¾ tsp. ground pepper
- ¾ tsp. salt

**The casserole:**

- 12 oz. chopped turkey sausage
- 4 thinly sliced green onions
- ¼ cup diced bell pepper
- ⅓ cup skim milk
- 6 large eggs
- 4 egg whites
- ¾ cup shredded cheddar cheese
- 16 oz. low-fat cottage cheese

**Directions**

**The crust:**

- Preheat the oven to 425°F. Lightly grease a 9×13-inch baking dish with 1 tbsp. olive oil and set aside.
- Squeeze excess moisture out of the potato with a kitchen towel or paper towel.

- Toss together the potatoes, the remaining olive oil, salt and pepper in a medium bowl until potatoes are well coated.
- Transfer the mixture to the greased baking dish; evenly press the mixture up the sides and on the bottom of the dish and bake for about 20 minutes or until golden brown on the edges.

**The casserole:**

- Reduce the oven heat to 375°F.
- In a large skillet, cook turkey sausage over medium-high heat for about 2 minutes or until it's almost cooked through.
- Add green onions and red bell pepper and continue cooking for 2 more minutes or until bell pepper is tender.
- Whisk together skim milk, eggs, egg whites, and the cheeses.
- Stir in turkey sausage mixture; pour over the potato crust and bake for about 50 minutes. Slightly cool and cut into 12 pieces. Enjoy!

# Yogurt Pancakes

Total time: 15 minutes

Prep time: 10 minutes

Cooking time: 5 minutes

Yield: 5 servings

**Ingredients**

- Whole-wheat pancake mix
- 1 cup yogurt
- 1 tbsp. baking powder
- 1 tbsp. baking soda
- 1 cup skimmed milk
- 3 whole eggs
- ½ tsp. extra virgin olive oil

**Directions**

- Combine together whole-wheat pancake mix, yogurt, baking powder, baking soda, skimmed milk and eggs in large bowl.
- Stir until well blended.
- Heat a pan oiled lightly with olive oil.
- Pour ¼ cup batter onto the heated pan and cook for about 2 minutes or until the surface of the pancake has some bubbles.
- Flip and continue cooking until the underside is browned.
- Serve the pancakes warm with a cup of fat-free milk or two tablespoons light maple syrup.

# Breakfast Stir Fry

Total time: 25 minutes

Prep time: 5 minutes

Cooking time: 20 minutes

Yield: 4 servings

**Ingredients**

- 1 tbsp. extra virgin olive oil
- 2 green peppers, sliced
- 2 small onions, finely chopped
- 4 tomatoes, chopped
- ½ tsp. sea salt
- 1 egg

**Directions**

- Heat olive oil in a medium-sized pan over medium-high heat.
- Add green pepper and sauté for about 2 minutes.
- Lower heat to medium and continue cooking, covered, for 3 more minutes.
- Stir in onion and cook for about 2 minutes or until brown.
- Stir in tomatoes and salt; cover and simmer to get a soft juicy mixture.
- In a bowl, beat the egg; drizzle over the tomato mixture and cook for about 1 minute. (Don't stir).
- Serve with chopped cucumbers, feta cheese and black olives for a great breakfast!

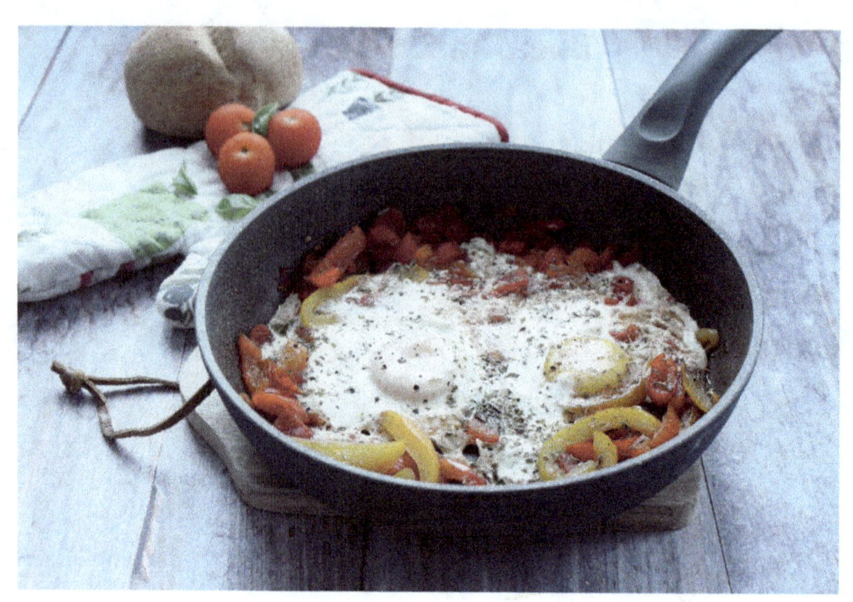

# MEDITERRANEAN LUNCH RECIPE

# Pecan Brown Butter Oat Triangles Recipe

## Ingredients

- ½ cup pecan halves
- ½ cup butter
- ¼ cup light corn syrup
- ½ cup packed light brown sugar
- 1/8 teaspoon salt
- 1 teaspoon vanilla extract
- 2 ½ cups rolled oats

## Preparation

- Preheat the oven to 350F. Line an 8- by an 8-inch baking dish with parchment (no greasing needed), or line with generously greased foil and set aside.

- Place pecans on a baking sheet and toast in the middle of the oven until they are 1 or 2 shades darker, 7 to 9 minutes, stirring once after 4 minutes. Watch carefully to prevent burning. Remove from the oven, pour into a small bowl and place nuts in the freezer to cool until they can be handled safely. Once they are cool, coarsely chop the pecans.

- In a 2-quart saucepan over medium-high heat, melt the butter while swirling the pan periodically. Adjust the heat to maintain gentle bubbling until foam turns a very light golden color and the liquid butter underneath begins to brown, 3 to 4 minutes. Continue to cook and swirl the pan until the liquid butter under the foam turns copper-colored, 2 to 3 minutes more. Remove the pan from the heat and stir in the corn syrup until dissolved. Stir in the brown sugar and salt and return to heat. Boil for 1 minute. Remove pan from heat again and stir in vanilla.

- Add oats and pecans to the saucepan and stir to coat. Pour the mixture into the prepared baking dish and spread evenly. Place a small piece of parchment paper or oiled foil on top of oats and press down firmly with your hand to flatten, paying attention to sides and corners. Use care: the mixture is still quite hot. Bake in the middle of the oven until the edges turn light golden brown, 13 to 15 minutes.
- Remove from the oven and place on a cooling rack for 15 minutes. Remove the whole bar from the pan by lifting the edges of the parchment paper and place it on a cutting board. While still warm, use a large chef's knife to cut the bar into 16 squares. Cut each square diagonally into 2 triangles (1 3/4 x 1 3/4 x 2 1/2-inch) to make 32 pieces. Cool completely, then store in an airtight container.

# Golden Pilaf

Yield: 6 servings

- 2 teaspoons olive oil
- 1 medium onion, chopped
- 1/4 cup golden raisins
- 1 cup long-grain rice
- 1/2 teaspoon turmeric
- 1/8 teaspoon cinnamon
- 1/8 teaspoon cardamom
- 2 cups low-sodium chicken or vegetable stock
- 1/4 cup pistachios, chopped
- 1/4 cup parsley, chopped

**Directions**

- In a 2-quart saucepan, heat the olive oil over medium-high heat. Add the onions and raisins and sauté for 3 minutes.
- Stir in the rice, turmeric, cinnamon, and cardamom and sauté for 1 minute. Add the stock, bring the mixture to a boil, and cover.
- Reduce the heat to a simmer for 15 to 18 minutes or until the liquid is fully absorbed.
- Meanwhile, toast the pistachios in small nonstick skillet for 1 minute or until fragrant. Add the pistachios and parsley to the cooked rice and serve.

Per serving: Calories 205 (From Fat 43); Fat 5g (Saturated 1g); Cholesterol 0mg; Sodium 48mg; Carbohydrate 36g (Dietary Fiber 2g); Protein 6g.

# Wild Rice Pilaf

- 2 cups wild rice, cooked
- 2 cups orzo, cooked
- 2 cups baby spinach leaves, chopped
- 1/4 cup kalamata olives, pitted
- 1/4 cup fresh dill, chopped
- 1/4 cup fresh parsley, chopped
- 1/4 cup olive oil
- Juice of 1 lemon
- 1 cup grape tomatoes, halved lengthwise
- Salt and pepper to taste
- 2 ounces feta cheese, crumbled

**Directions**

- In a large bowl, combine the rice, orzo, spinach, olives, dill, and olive oil. Toss to coat.
- Add the lemon juice and gently stir in the tomatoes and parsley. Season with salt and pepper to taste. Top with the cheese and serve.

# Moroccan Couscous

- 1-1/2 cups vegetable stock
- Zest and juice of 1 orange
- 1/3 cup chopped dates
- 1/3 cup chopped dried apricots
- 1/3 cup golden raisins
- 1/4 teaspoon ground cinnamon
- 1/2 teaspoon ground cumin
- 1/4 teaspoon coriander
- 1/2 teaspoon ground ginger
- 1/2 teaspoon turmeric
- 2 cups dry plain or whole-wheat couscous
- 1 tablespoon butter
- 1/2 cup slivered almonds, toasted
- 1/4 cup mint, chopped
- Salt to taste

**Directions**

- In a medium saucepan, bring the stock to a boil. Add the orange juice and zest, dates, apricots, raisins, spices, and couscous.
- Cover and remove the pan from the heat.
- Allow the couscous to absorb the liquid, about 15 minutes. If your couscous is too dry, add a bit of water, cover, and wait 5 minutes; repeat until the couscous is the desired consistency.

- Uncover, add the butter, and mix well. Stir in the almonds and mint and season with salt to taste before serving.

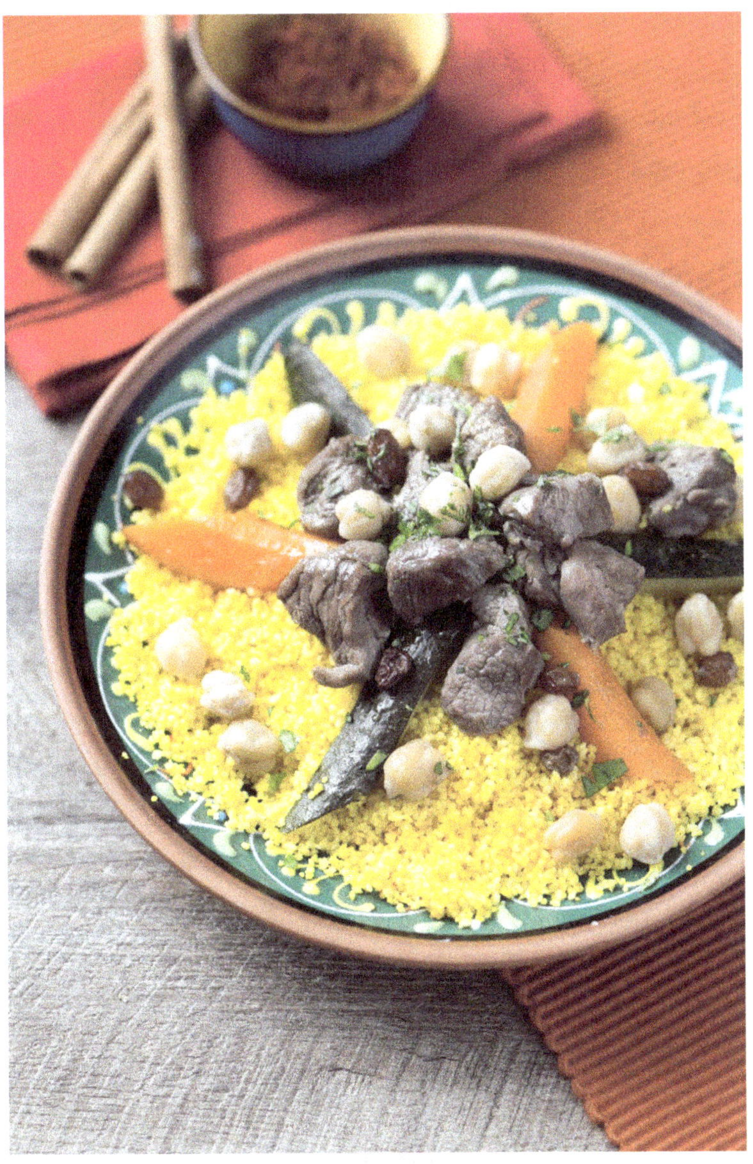

# Couscous with Tomatoes and Cucumbers

- 2 cups water
- 1 cup whole-wheat couscous
- 1/2 teaspoon coriander
- 2 Roma or plum tomatoes, chopped
- 1 small cucumber, seeded and chopped
- 1/2 medium red onion, chopped
- One 14.5-ounce can chickpeas, drained and rinsed
- 1/2 cup fresh mint, chopped
- 1/3 cup lemon juice
- 1 tablespoon olive oil
- Salt and pepper to taste

**Directions**

- In a medium saucepan, bring the water to a boil.
- Stir in the couscous and coriander, cover, and remove from the heat. Allow the couscous to absorb the liquid completely, about 15 minutes.
- Combine the cooked couscous with the tomatoes, cucumber, onions, chickpeas, and mint in a large bowl.
- Whisk together the lemon juice and olive oil, pour the mixture over the couscous salad, and stir well.
- Cover and refrigerate for at least 2 hours. Serve.

# Charcuterie Bistro Lunch Box

**Ingredients**

- 1 slice prosciutto
- 1 mozzarella stick, halved
- 2 breadsticks, halved
- 2 dates
- ½ cup grapes
- 2 large radishes, halved or 4 slices English cucumber (1/4-inch)

**Directions**

- Cut prosciutto in half lengthwise, then wrap a slice around each portion of cheese. Arrange the wrapped cheese, breadsticks, dates, grapes and radishes (or cucumber) in a 4-cup divided sealable container. Keep refrigerated until ready to eat.

# Mediterranean Chicken Quinoa Bowl

## Ingredients

- 1 pound boneless, skinless chicken breasts, trimmed
- ¼ teaspoon salt
- ¼ teaspoon ground pepper
- 1 7-ounce jar roasted red peppers, rinsed
- ¼ cup slivered almonds
- 4 tablespoons extra-virgin olive oil, divided
- 1 small clove garlic, crushed
- 1 teaspoon paprika
- ½ teaspoon ground cumin
- ¼ teaspoon crushed red pepper (Optional)
- 2 cups cooked quinoa
- ¼ cup pitted Kalamata olives, chopped
- ¼ cup finely chopped red onion
- 1 cup diced cucumber
- ¼ cup crumbled feta cheese
- 2 tablespoons finely chopped fresh parsley

## Directions

- Position a rack in upper third of oven; preheat broiler to high. Line a rimmed baking sheet with foil.
- Sprinkle chicken with salt and pepper and place on the prepared baking sheet. Broil, turning once, until an instant-read thermometer inserted in the thickest part reads 165 degrees F, 14 to 18 minutes. Transfer the chicken to a clean cutting board and slice or shred.

- Meanwhile, place peppers, almonds, 2 tablespoons oil, garlic, paprika, cumin and crushed red pepper (if using) in a mini food processor. Puree until fairly smooth.

- Combine quinoa, olives, red onion and the remaining 2 tablespoons oil in a medium bowl.

- To serve, divide the quinoa mixture among 4 bowls and top with equal amounts of cucumber, the chicken and the red pepper sauce. Sprinkle with feta and parsley.

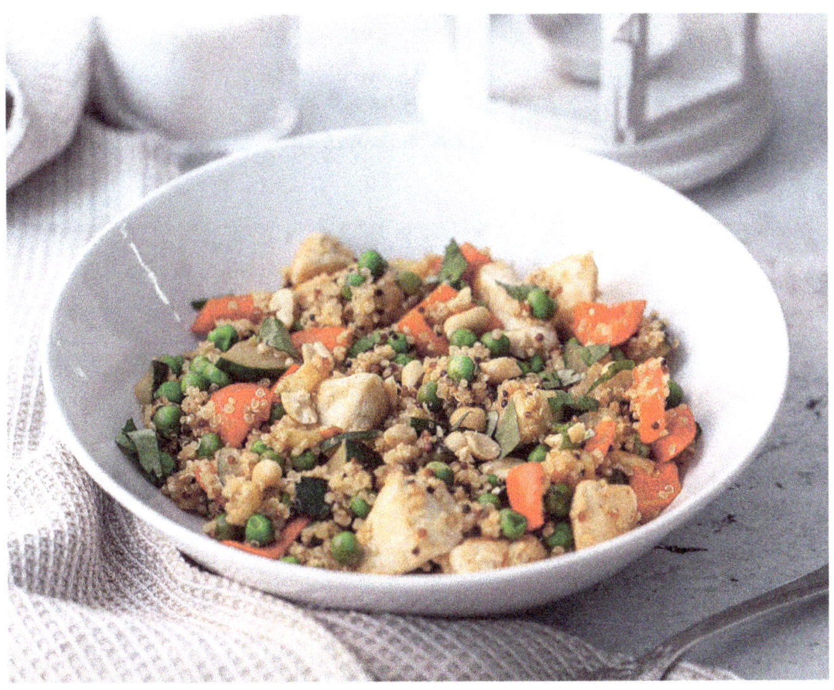

# MEDITERRANEAN

# SALAD RECIPES

# Italian Bread Salad

Total time: 2 hours 30 minutes

Prep time: 25 minutes, plus 2 hours Refrigerator time

Cook time: 5 minutes

Yield: 4 servings

**Ingredients**

- 3 tbsp. freshly squeezed lemon juice
- 2 tbsp. extra virgin olive oil
- Sea salt
- Freshly ground pepper
- 1 red onion, halved and sliced
- 1 bulb fennel, stalks removed and sliced
- 1 peeled English cucumber, sliced
- 1 ½ pounds diced tomatoes
- ⅓ cup pitted Kalamata olives, halved
- 4 slices whole-wheat country bread
- 1 garlic clove, peeled and halved
- 4 ounces shaved ricotta salata cheese
- ½ cup fresh basil leaves

**Directions**

- Whisk together lemon juice and extra virgin olive oil in a large bowl; season with sea salt and black pepper.
- Stir in onion, fennel, cucumber, tomatoes, and olives; toss to combine and refrigerate for about 2 hours.

- When ready, heat your broiler with the rack positioned 4 inches from heat and toast the bread on a baking sheet for about 2 minutes per side or until lightly browned.
- Transfer the toasted bread to a work surface and rub with the cut garlic and cut it into 2-inch pieces.
- Divide the bread among four shallow bowls and top with the tomato salad; sprinkle with cheese and basil to serve.

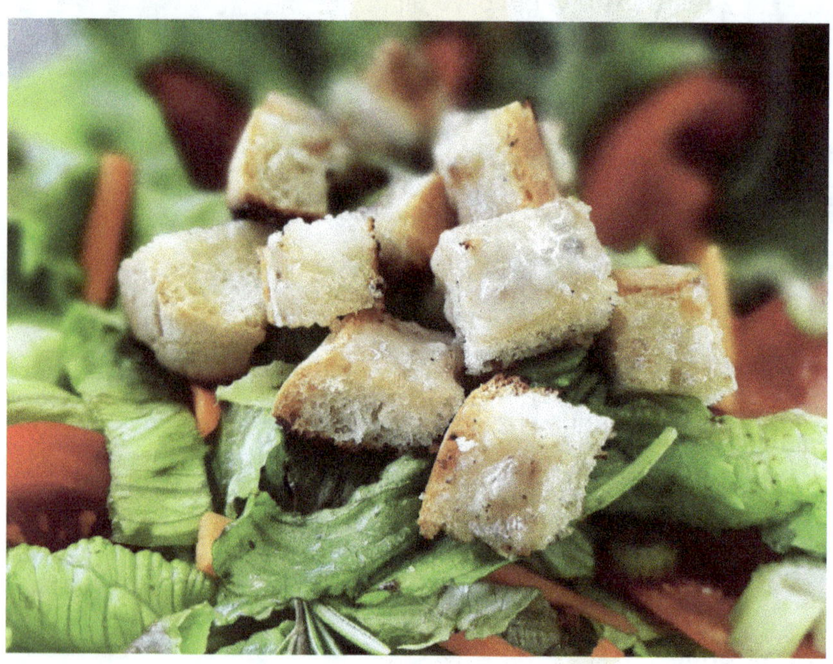

# Bulgur Salad

Total time: 30 minutes

Prep time: 10 minutes

Cook time: 20 minutes

Yield: 4 servings

**Ingredients**

- 1 tbsp. unsalted butter
- 2 tbsp. extra virgin olive oil, divided
- 2 cups bulgur
- 4 cups water
- ¼ tsp. sea salt
- 1 medium cucumber, deseeded and chopped
- ¼ cup dill, chopped
- 1 handful black olives, pitted and chopped
- 2 tsp. red wine vinegar

**Directions**

- Place a saucepan over medium heat and add 1 tbsp. of butter and 1 tbsp. of olive oil.
- Toast the bulgur in the oil until it turns golden brown and starts to crackle.
- Add 4 cups of water to the saucepan and season with the salt.
- Cover the saucepan and simmer until all the water gets absorbed for about 20 minutes.
- In a mixing bowl, combine the chopped cucumber with dill, olives, red wine vinegar and the remaining olive oil.

- Serve this over the bulgur.

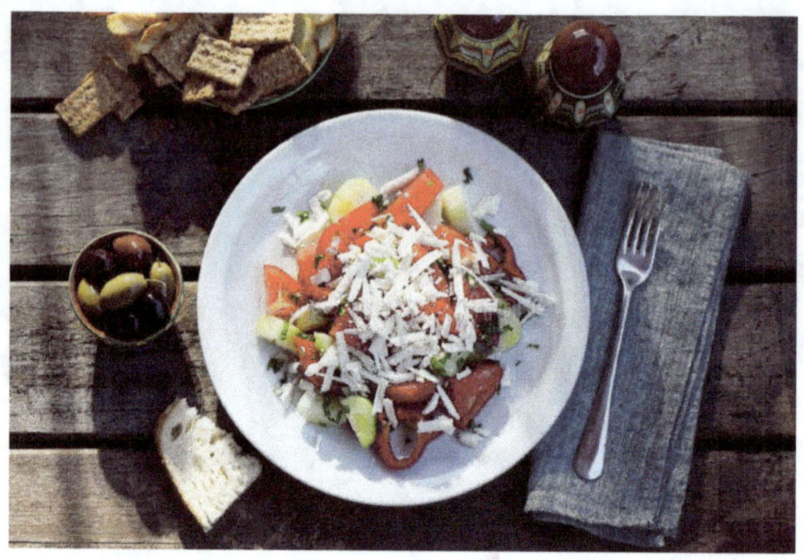

# Greek Salad

Total time: 20 minutes

Prep time: 20 minutes

Cook time: 0 minutes

Yield: 4 servings

**Ingredients**

- Juice of 1 lemon
- 6 tbsp. extra virgin olive oil
- Black pepper to taste, ground
- 1 tsp. oregano, dried
- 1 head romaine lettuce, washed, dried and chopped
- 1 red bell pepper, chopped
- 1 green bell pepper, chopped
- 1 cucumber, sliced
- 2 tomatoes, chopped
- 1 cup feta cheese, crumbled
- 1 red onion, thinly sliced
- 1 can black olives, pitted

**Directions**

- Whisk together the lemon juice, olive oil, pepper and oregano in a small bowl.
- In a large bowl, combine the lettuce, bell peppers, cucumber, tomatoes, cheese and onion.
- Pour the salad dressing into this bowl and toss until evenly coated with the dressing, then serve.

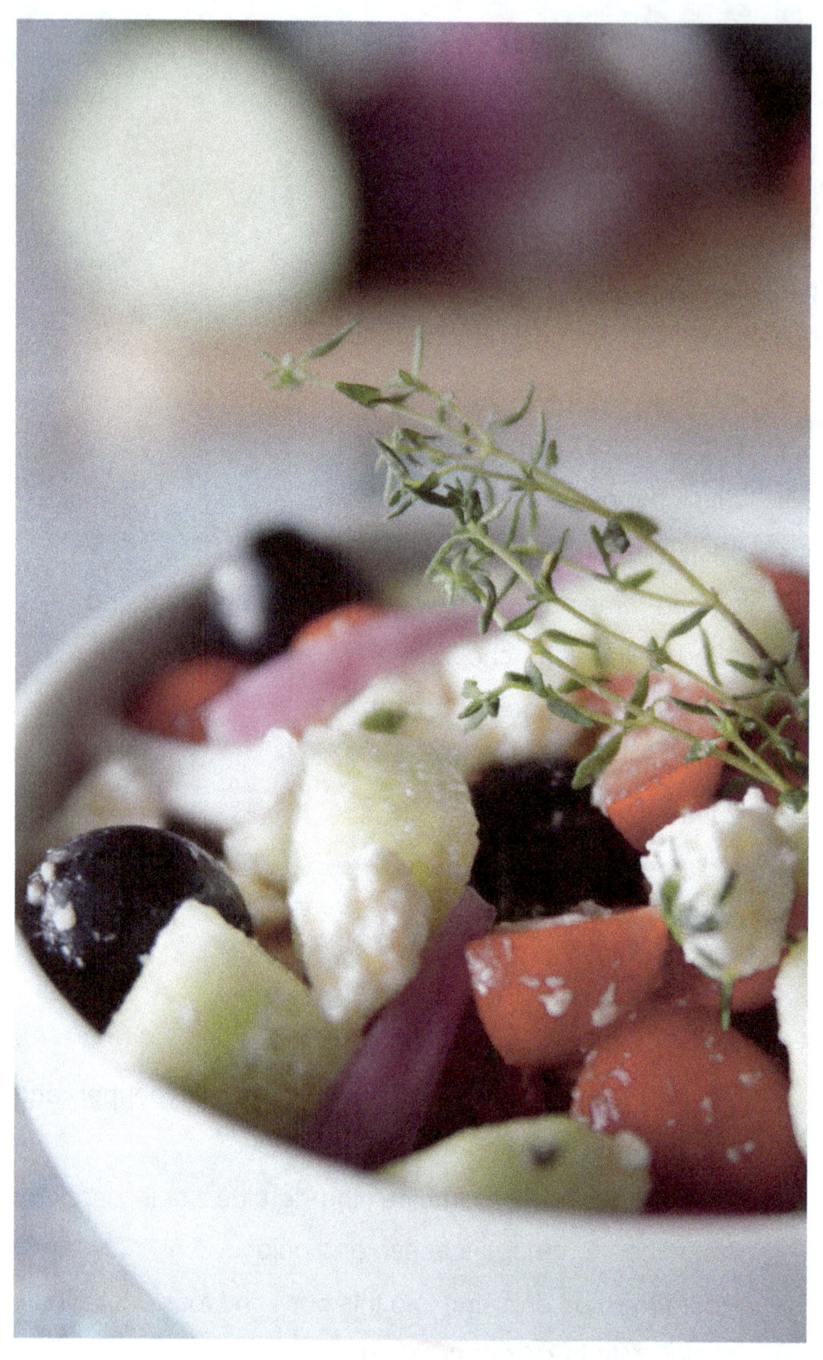

# MEDITERRANEAN POULTRY RECIPES

# Warm Chicken Avocado Salad

Total time: 35 minutes

Prep time: 15 minutes

Cook time: 20 minutes

Yield: 4 servings

**Ingredients**

- 2 tbsp. extra virgin olive oil, divided
- 500g chicken breast fillets
- 1 large avocado, peeled, diced
- 2 garlic cloves, sliced
- 1 tsp. ground turmeric
- 3 tsp. ground cumin
- 1 small head broccoli, chopped
- 1 large carrot, diced
- 1/3 cup currants
- 1 1/2 cups chicken stock
- 1 1/2 cups couscous
- Pinch of sea salt

**Directions**

- In a large frying pan set over medium heat, heat 1 tablespoon extra virgin olive oil; add chicken and cook for about 6 minutes per side or until cooked through; transfer to a plate and keep warm.

- In the meantime, combine currants and couscous in a heatproof bowl; stir in boiling stock and set aside, covered, for at least 5 minutes or until liquid is absorbed.

- With a fork, separate the grains.
- Add the remaining oil to a frying pan and add carrots; cook, stirring, for about 1 minute.
- Stir in broccoli for about 1 minute; stir in garlic, turmeric, and cumin.
- Cook for about 1 minute more and remove the pan from heat.
- Slice the chicken into small slices and add to the broccoli mixture; toss to combine; season with sea salt and serve with the avocado sprinkled on top.

# Chicken Stew

Total time: 35 minutes

Prep time: 20 minutes

Cook time: 15 minutes

Yield: 4 servings

**Ingredients**

- 1 tbsp. extra virgin olive oil
- 3 chicken breast halves (8 ounces each), boneless, skinless, cut into small pieces
- Sea salt
- Freshly ground pepper
- 1 medium onion, sliced
- 4 garlic cloves, sliced
- ½ tsp. dried oregano
- 1 ½ pounds escarole, ends trimmed, chopped
- 1 cup whole-wheat couscous, cooked
- 1 (28 ounces) can whole peeled tomatoes, pureed

**Directions**

- In a large heavy pot or Dutch oven, heat extra virgin olive oil over medium high heat.
- Rub chicken with sea salt and pepper.
- In batches, cook chicken in olive oil, tossing occasionally, for about 5 minutes or until browned; transfer to a plate and set aside.

- Add onion, garlic and oregano, tomatoes, sea salt and pepper to the pot and cook for about 10 minutes or until onion is lightly browned.
- Add the chicken and cook, covered for about 4 minutes or until opaque.
- Fill the pot with escarole and cook for about 4 minutes or until tender.
- Serve the chicken stew over couscous.

# Chicken with Roasted Vegetables

Total time: 55 minutes

Prep time: 15 minutes

Cook time: 40 minutes

Yield: 2 servings

**Ingredients**

- 1 large zucchini, diagonally sliced
- 250g baby new potatoes, sliced
- 6 firm plum tomatoes, halved
- 1 red onion, cut into wedges
- 1 yellow pepper, seeded and cut into chunks
- 12 black olives, pitted
- 2 chicken breast fillets, skinless, boneless
- 1 rounded tbsp. green pesto
- 3 tbsp. extra virgin olive oil

**Directions**

- Preheat your oven to 400ºF.
- Spread zucchini, potatoes, tomatoes, onion, and pepper in a roasting pan and scatter with olives.
- Season with sea salt and black pepper.
- Cut each chicken breast into four pieces and arrange them on top of the vegetables.
- In a small bowl, combine pesto and extra virgin olive oil and spread over the chicken. Cover with foil and cook in preheated oven for about 30 minutes.

- Uncover the pan and return to oven; cook for about 10 minutes more or until chicken is cooked through.
- Enjoy!

41

# Grilled Chicken with Olive Relish

Total time: 21 minutes

Prep time: 15 minutes

Cook time: 6 minutes

Yield: 4 servings

**Ingredients**

- 4 chicken breast halves, boneless, skinless
- ¾ cup extra virgin olive oil, divided
- Sea salt
- Freshly ground black pepper
- 2 tbsp. capers, rinsed, chopped
- 1 ½ cups green olives, rinsed, pitted, and chopped
- ¼ cup lightly toasted almonds, chopped
- 1 small clove garlic, mashed with sea salt
- 1 ½ tsp. chopped fresh thyme
- 2 ½ tsp. grated lemon zest
- 2 tbsp. chopped fresh parsley

**Directions**

- Heat grill to high heat.
- Place 1 chicken breast on one side of a plastic wrap and drizzle with about 1 teaspoon of extra virgin olive oil and fold the wrap over the chicken.
- Pound the chicken with a heavy sauté pan or a meat mallet to about ½ inch thick.
- Repeat the process with the remaining chicken and discard the plastic wrap.

- Sprinkle chicken with sea salt and pepper and coat with about 2 tablespoons extra virgin olive oil; set aside.
- In the meantime, combine ½ cup extra virgin olive oil, capers, olives, almonds, garlic, thyme, lemon zest and parsley in a medium bowl.
- Grill the chicken for about 3 minutes per side and transfer to a cutting board.
- Let cool a bit and cut into ½-inch-thick slices.
- Arrange the chicken slices on four plates and spoon over the relish.
- Serve immediately.

# MEDITERRANEAN SEAFOOD RECIPES

# Grilled Tuna

Total time: 1 hour 16 minutes

Prep time: 10 minutes

Chill time: 1 hour

Cook time: 6 minutes

Yield: 4 servings

**Ingredients**

- 4 tuna steaks, 1 inch thick
- 3 tbsp. extra virgin oil
- ½ cup hickory wood chips, soaked
- Sea salt
- Freshly ground black pepper
- Juice of 1 lime

**Directions**

- Place tuna and the olive oil in a zip lock plastic bag, seal and refrigerate for an hour.
- Prepare a charcoal or gas grill.
- When using a coal grill, scatter a handful of hickory wood chips when the coals are hot for added flavor.
- Lightly grease the grill grate.
- Season the tuna with salt and pepper and cook on the grill for about 6 minutes, turning only once.
- Transfer to a plate.
- Drizzle the lime juice over the fish and serve immediately.

# Easy Fish Dish

Total time: 45 minutes

Prep time: 15 minutes

Cook time: 30 minutes

Yields: 4 servings

**Ingredients**

- 4 fillets halibut (6 ounces)
- 1 tbsp. Greek seasoning
- 1 tbsp. lemon juice
- ¼ cup olive oil
- ¼ cup capers
- 1 jar (5 ounce) pitted Kalamata olives
- 1 chopped onion
- 1 large tomato, chopped
- A pinch of freshly ground black pepper   A pinch of salt

**Directions**

- Preheat your oven to 250°F.
- Arrange the halibut fillets onto an aluminum foil sheet and sprinkle with Greek seasoning.
- In a bowl, combine together lemon juice, olive oil, capers, olives, onion, tomato, salt and pepper; spoon the mixture over the fillets and fold the edges of the foil to seal.
- Place the folded foil onto a baking sheet and bake for about 40 minutes or until the fish flakes easily when touched with a fork.

# Salmon Bean Stir-Fry

Total time: 20 minutes

Prep time: 10 minutes

Cook time: 10 minutes

Yield: 4 servings

**Ingredients**

- 1g crushed red pepper
- 2.5g cornstarch
- 5ml rice wine
- 7.5ml black bean-garlic sauce
- 7.5ml rice vinegar
- 30ml cup water
- 5ml canola oil
- 100g salmon, skinned, cubed
- 10g scallions, sliced
- 90g bean sprouts

**Directions**

- In a bowl, whisk together crushed red pepper, cornstarch, rice wine, bean-garlic sauce, vinegar and water until well combined.
- Add oil to skillet set over medium heat.
- Stir in fish and cook for about 2 minutes.
- Stir in the sauce mixture, scallions and sprouts.
- Cook for about 3 minutes or until the sprouts are tender and cooked down.

# Mediterranean Flounder

Total time: 40 minutes

Prep time: 10 minutes

Cook time: 30 minutes

Yield: 4 servings

**Ingredients**

- 5 Roma tomatoes
- 2 tbsp. extra virgin olive oil
- ½ onion, chopped
- 2 garlic cloves, chopped
- 1 pinch Italian seasoning
- 1 lb. flounder/tilapia/halibut
- 4 tbsp. capers
- 24 Kalamata olives, pitted and chopped
- 1 tsp. freshly squeezed lemon juice
- ¼ cup white wine
- 6 leaves fresh basil, chopped; divided
- 3 tbsp. Parmesan cheese

**Directions**

- Preheat your oven to 425ºF.
- Plunge the tomatoes into boiling water and immediately transfer them into a bowl of ice water; peel the skins and chop them
- Add extra virgin olive oil to a skillet set over medium heat and sauté onions until translucent.

- Stir in garlic, Italian seasoning, and tomatoes and cook until tomatoes are tender.
- Stir in wine, lemon juice, capers, olives, and half of basil.
- Lower heat and stir in Parmesan cheese; cook for about 15 minutes or until the mixture is bubbly and hot.
- Place fish in a baking dish and cover with the sauce; bake in the preheated oven for about 20 minutes or until fish is cooked through.

# MEDITERRANEAN MEAT, BEEF AND PORK RECIPES

# Healthy Lamb Burgers

Total time: 40 minutes

Prep time: 10 minutes, plus 20 minutes resting time

Cook time: 10 minutes

Yield: 4 servings

**Ingredients**

- 1 tbsp. extra virgin olive oil
- 1 lb. lean ground lamb
- 2 tbsp. yogurt cheese
- ⅛ tsp. ground allspice
- ½ cup cilantro leaves, chopped
- 1 small egg white
- 1 shallot, finely chopped
- 2 cloves garlic, chopped
- 2 tsp. fresh ginger, minced
- 1 red chili pepper, chopped
- ⅛ tsp. ground cumin
- 4 cardamom seeds
- ⅛ tsp. black pepper
- ¼ tsp. sea salt
- spray olive oil
- 4 whole-wheat hamburger buns

**Directions**

- Mix together all the ingredients except spray olive oil and buns, and refrigerate for at least 20 minutes.
- Preheat your oven to 400° F.

- Heat extra virgin olive oil in a large nonstick skillet over medium heat.
- In the meantime, form lamb mixture into 4 burgers.
- Sear burgers in prepared pan for about 1 minute; transfer the pan to the preheated oven and cook for about 5 minutes, turn burgers over and cook for about 3 minutes more.

# Herb-Maple Crusted Steak

Total time: 25 minutes

Prep time: 15 minutes

Cook time: 10 minutes

Yield: 4 servings

**Ingredients**

- 3 tbsp. rosemary
- 3 tbsp. fresh tarragon
- 3 tbsp. chives
- 3 tbsp. chopped oregano
- 4 tbsp. parsley
- 3 tbsp. maple syrup
- 4 (4 ounce) ribeye steaks, trimmed
- ½ tsp. sea salt
- ¼ tsp. black pepper
- spray olive oil

**Directions**

- Preheat your oven to 450°F.
- Heat a nonstick skillet in the oven.
- In the meantime, combine the minced herbs on a plate
- Add maple syrup to a separate bowl.
- Season steak with sea salt and pepper and dip into the maple syrup; turn to coat well.
- Dip the steak into the herbs and turn to coat well. Repeat with the remaining steak.

- Remove the skillet from oven and spray with extra virgin olive oil; add steaks to the pan and turn until well seared.
- Return to oven and cook for about 4 minutes, turn and cook the other side for about 6 minutes more.

# Tenderloin with Blue Cheese Butter

Total time: 30 minutes

Prep time: 15 minutes

Cook time: 15 minutes

Yield: 2 servings

**Ingredients**

- ⅛ tsp. black pepper
- 1 small shallot, minced
- 1 tsp. unsalted butter
- 2 tbsp. chopped parsley
- 2 tsp. blue cheese
- Extra virgin olive oil spray
- 2 4-ounce beef tenderloin filets
- ¼ tsp. sea salt

**Directions**

- In a blender, blend together pepper, shallot, butter, parsley and blue cheese until very smooth.
- Preheat your oven to 450°F.
- Place a nonstick skillet in oven and spray with extra virgin olive oil.
- Season beef with sea salt and place in the pan; cook for about 7 minutes, turn over and cook the other side for about 4 minutes more.
- Transfer the meat to a plate and top with seasoned butter to serve.

# Green Curry Beef

Total time: 1 hour, 20 minutes

Prep time: 10 minutes

Resting time: 30 minutes

Cook time: 40 minutes

Yield: 3 servings

**Ingredients**

- 1 tbsp. extra virgin olive oil
- ½ cup chopped parsley
- 1 cup cilantro leaves
- 1 white onion, chopped
- 1 fresh Thai green chili, chopped
- 2 cloves garlic, thinly sliced
- ¼ tsp. turmeric
- ½ tsp. ground cumin
- 2 tbsp. lime juice
- ¼ tsp. sea salt
- Black pepper
- 16 ounces beef top round, cut into small pieces
- 1 can light coconut milk
- 1/4 tsp. turmeric
- 1/2 tsp. ground cumin
- 1/4 tsp. sea salt

**Directions**

**Green curry paste:**

- In a food processor or blender, combine extra virgin olive oil, parsley, cilantro, onion, chili pepper, garlic, turmeric, cumin, lime juice, sea salt, and pepper; process until very smooth.
- Combine beef and green curry paste in a bowl; toss to coat.
- Refrigerate for at least 30 minutes.
- When ready, heat a large skillet over medium high heat and add beef along with the green curry sauce.
- Lower heat and stir for about 10 minutes or until the meat is browned on the outside.
- Stir in coconut milk and cook for about 30 minutes or until the sauce is thick.
- Serve immediately.

# VEGETARIAN AND LEGUMES MEDITERRANEAN RECIPES

# Chorizo Pilau

Total time: 50 minutes

Prep time: 10 minutes

Cook time: 40 minutes

Yield: 4 servings

**Ingredients**

- 1 tbsp. extra virgin olive oil

- 1 large red onion, thinly sliced

- ¼ kg baby cooking chorizo, sliced

- 4 garlic cloves, minced

- 1 tsp. paprika, smoked

- 1 can tomatoes, chopped

- ¼ kg basmati rice

- 4 garlic cloves, minced

- ½ liter stock

- 1 small bunch parsley, chopped

- Zest of 1 lemon, peeled in thick strips and the remainder wedged   2 bay leaves, fresh

**Directions**

- Place a thick saucepan on medium heat and pour in the oil.

- Add the onion and let it cook until golden brown for about 6 minutes.

- Push the onions to one side of the pan, pour in the chorizo and let it cook until it starts releasing some of its oils.

- The garlic and paprika are next.

- Stir for 2 minutes, then add the tomatoes and let cook for 5 minutes.
- Pour in the rice, lemon zest, bay leaves and stock.
- Stir everything in the pan and bring to a boil.
- Cover the pan and simmer for 12 minutes.
- Turn of the heat, take the lid off and cover the pan with foil, then put the lid back on and let it sit for about 15 minutes.
- Stir in the parsley and serve with lemon wedges. (Squeezing in the lemons gives the dish an amazing taste.)

# Pasta with Raisins, Garbanzos, and Spinach

Total time: 40 minutes

Prep time: 15 minutes

Cook time: 25 minutes

Yield: 6 servings

**Ingredients**

- 8 ounces farfalle (bow tie) pasta
- 2 tbsp. extra virgin olive oil
- 4 garlic cloves, crushed
- ½ cup chicken broth (unsalted)
- ½ (19 ounces) can rinsed and drained garbanzos
- 4 cups chopped fresh spinach
- ½ cup golden raisins
- 2 tbsp. Parmesan cheese
- Cracked black peppercorns

**Directions**

- Fill a pot ¾ full with salted water; bring to a rolling boil over high heat.
- Add pasta and cook for about 12 minutes or until al dente; drain and set aside.
- Heat extra virgin olive oil in a large skillet and sauté garlic until fragrant; add chicken broth and garbanzo beans and stir until warmed through.
- Stir in spinach and raisins and cook for about 3 minutes or until spinach is wilted.

- Divide pasta among plates and top each with about 1/6 of sauce, peppercorns and Parmesan.
- Serve right away.

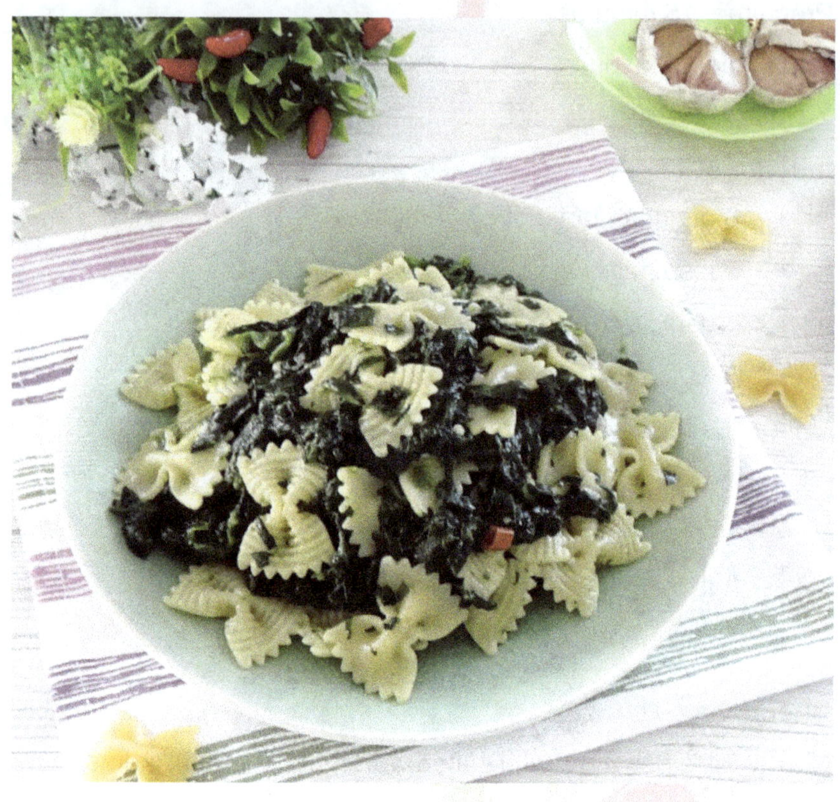

# Eggplant Steak with Black Olives, Roasted Peppers, Chickpeas and Feta Cheese

Total time: 30 minutes

Prep time: 20 minutes

Cook time: 10 minutes

Yield: 4 servings

**Balsamic Marinade**

- 2 cloves garlic, minced
- 1 tbsp. low-sodium tamari
- 1 tbsp. balsamic vinegar
- ¼ tsp. freshly ground black pepper
- 2 tbsp. extra virgin olive oil

**Eggplant Steaks**

- 1 large eggplant, about 1 lb.
- ¼ lb. crumbled feta cheese
- 2 roasted red peppers, diced
- 1 ½ cups chickpeas, drained
- 4 tsp. balsamic vinegar
- Pinch of oregano
- ½ cup pitted black olives
- Sea salt
- Freshly ground black pepper
- 4 (6½-inch round) pita breads
- Fresh oregano, for garnish

**Directions:**

**Make marinade:**

In a bowl, combine marinade ingredients, gradually stirring in extra virgin olive oil until well combined.

* Set aside.
* Preheat your broiler or grill.
* Cut the eggplant into 4 ¼-inch-thick slices, lengthwise to look like steaks.
* Brush the eggplant slices with the marinade and broil or grill for about 2 minutes per side or until tender.
* Transfer the grilled eggplants to the plates, one on each.
* In a small bowl, combine feta, red peppers, chickpeas, oregano and black olives; season with sea salt and ground black pepper.
* Stir until well blended; stir in some marinade.
* Grill or toast pita bread and cut into wedges; set aside.
* Ladle about 2 scoops of the olive-pepper mixture onto eggplant "steak" and drizzle with balsamic vinegar.
* Add a few pita bread wedges and garnish with oregano sprigs.
* Repeat with the remaining ingredients and serve immediately.

# Tomato and Spinach Pasta

Total time: 35 minutes

Prep time: 10 minutes

Cook time: 25 minutes

**Ingredients**

- 100g whole-wheat pasta
- 7.5ml extra virgin olive oil
- ½ onion, sliced
- 60g can tomatoes, drained
- 60g frozen spinach
- ⅓ cup crumbled feta cheese
- 1g salt
- 1g ground pepper

**Directions**

- Follow package instructions to cook pasta in a pot of boiling water until al dente.
- In the meantime, add oil to a skillet set over medium heat; stir in onion and sauté for 3 minutes. Stir in tomatoes and simmer for about 10 minutes.
- Add spinach and cook until heated through.
- Drain the cooked pasta and toss with the sauce until well coated.
- Season with salt and pepper and serve topped with feta.

# MEDITERRANEAN DESSERTS

# **TIRAMISU**

Serves 10

- 3 large eggs, separated
- 1⁄8 teaspoon nutmeg
- 1⁄4 cup sugar, divided
- 1 cup mascarpone cheese
- 1⁄2 cup strong black coffee, freshly made 6 tablespoon Marsala or coffee liqueur
- 16 ladyfinger cookies, divided
- 2 tablespoons cocoa powder

**Directions**

- In a medium bowl, whisk egg yolks, nutmeg, and 2 tablespoons of sugar until the mixture has thickened. Stir in the mascarpone. In another medium bowl, beat the egg whites until they form stiff peaks. Gently fold the mascarpone-egg mixture into the egg whites. Set it aside.
- In a medium bowl, add the remaining sugar, coffee, and Marsala. Stir the mixture until the sugar is dissolved. Dip eight ladyfingers (one at a time) into the coffee mixture for 1 second, and then place it on a small baking dish. Don't leave the ladyfingers in the coffee for more than a second or they will be mushy.
- Spread half of the mascarpone filling over the ladyfingers. Dip the remaining ladyfingers (one at a time) in the coffee mixture for 1 second, and then place them in the dish over the filling. Spread the remaining mascarpone filling over

the ladyfingers. Cover the tiramisu and refrigerate it for 8 hours or overnight.

- Sprinkle the dessert with cocoa powder before serving. Serve it cool or at room temperature.

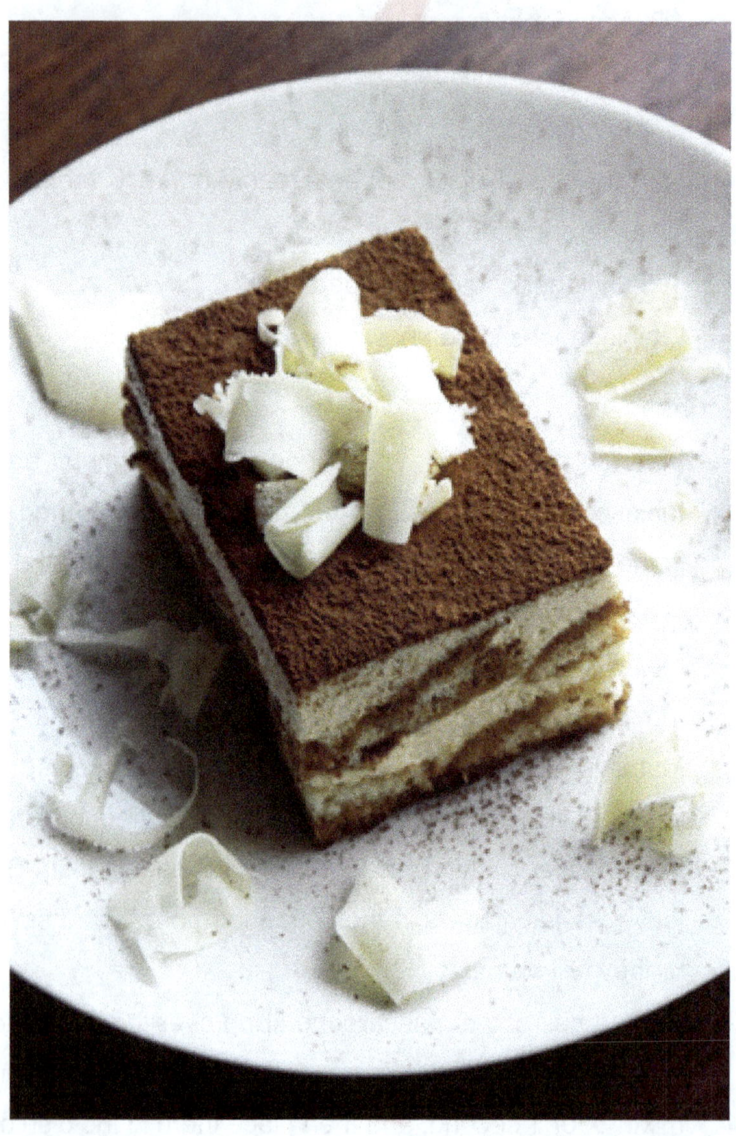

# EKMEK KATAIFI

Serves 10

- 1 cup sugar
- 1 cup water
- 2 (2-inch) strips lemon peel, pith removed
- 1 tablespoon fresh lemon juice
- 1⁄2 cup plus
- 1 tablespoon unsalted butter, melted and divided
- 1⁄2 pound frozen kataifi pastry, thawed, at room temperature
- 21⁄2 cups whole milk
- 1⁄2 teaspoon ground mastiha
- 2 large eggs
- 1⁄4 cup fine semolina
- 1 teaspoon of cornstarch
- 1⁄4 cup sugar
- 1⁄2 cup sweetened coconut flakes 1 cup whipping cream
- 1 teaspoon vanilla extract
- 1 teaspoon powdered milk
- 3 tablespoons confectioners' sugar
- 1⁄2 cup chopped unsalted pistachios

**Directions**

- Put the sugar, water, lemon peel, and lemon juice in a medium pot over medium-high heat. Bring the mixture to a boil, and then reduce the heat to medium-low and cook for

10 minutes. Allow the syrup to cool to room temperature and reserve.

- Preheat the oven to 350°F. Grease a 9" × 5" loaf pan with 1 tablespoon of butter. In a large bowl, add the kataifi (untangle first) and pour the remaining butter over it. Toss the kataifi in the butter to coat it and then add it to the pan. Bake the pastry on the middle rack of the oven for 30 minutes or until golden. Remove the pan from the oven and immediately ladle the reserved syrup over the kataifi. Allow the kataifi to cool to room temperature.

- Heat the milk and mastiha in a medium pot over medium-high heat until the milk is scalded (just before boiling). Immediately reduce the temperature to medium-low to keep milk warm. In a large bowl, whisk the eggs, semolina, cornstarch, and sugar. Slowly whisk a ladle of the milk mixture into the eggs. Add two more ladles, one at a time.

- Transfer the egg mixture into the pot with the milk, on medium heat. Stir until it thickens and has the consistency of custard. Stir in the coconut. Remove pot from the heat, and cover the surface with plastic wrap so it doesn't form a crust. Cool to room temperature.

- Spread the custard over the kataifi. Refrigerate for 8 hours or overnight to set. Unmold the kataifi by running a knife around the edges of the pan and flipping the pan over a serving plate. Invert the kataifi on the plate so the custard is facing up.

- In a large bowl, whip the cream until it forms soft peaks. Add the vanilla, powdered milk, and confectioners' sugar.

Resume whipping the cream until it forms stiff peaks. Spread the whipped cream over the custard, and top with the pistachios. Serve immediately.

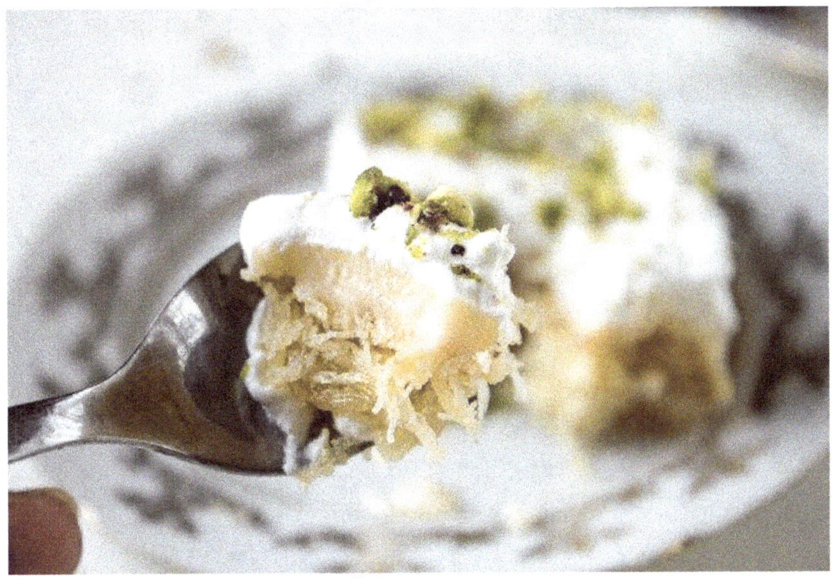

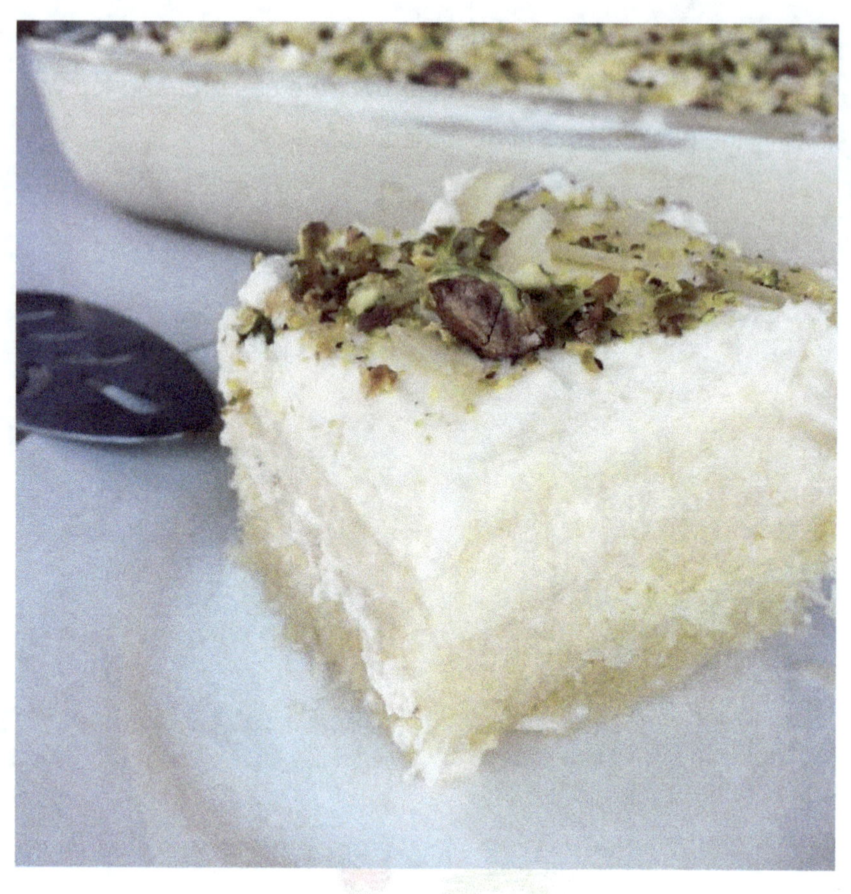

# PORTOKALOPITA (ORANGE PHYLLO PIE)

Serves 16

- 2 cups sugar, divided
- 2 cups water
- 2 large oranges, sliced
- 1/2 cup plus 1 tablespoon unsalted butter, melted and divided 1 package phyllo, thawed, at room temperature
- 2 teaspoons ground cinnamon
- 5 large eggs
- 2 tablespoons grated orange zest
- 1 teaspoon vanilla extract
- 1 tablespoon orange liqueur
- 1/8 teaspoon salt
- 11/2 teaspoons baking powder
- 11/2 cups extra-virgin olive oil
- 1 cup plain yogurt
- 1/2 cup raisins

**Directions**

- Heat 1 cup of sugar and the water in a medium pot over medium-high heat until it boils, and then reduce the heat to medium-low. Add the orange slices, and cook for 30–40 minutes or until the oranges soften and begin to look translucent. Remove the orange slices and discard them. Allow the syrup to cool to room temperature and reserve it.

- Preheat the oven to 350°F. Brush the bottom and sides of a 13" × 9" baking pan with 1 tablespoon of butter. Open the phyllo package, and cover sheets with a slightly damp tea towel so they don't dry out. In a small bowl, combine 1⁄2 cup of sugar and the cinnamon.

- Brush a phyllo sheet with melted butter, and sprinkle the surface with some of the cinnamon-sugar. Loosely fold about 1 inch of phyllo from the bottom over the cinnamon sugar and lightly pinch the right and left ends. Continue to loosely fold, over and under so it looks like ruffled curtains, and lightly pinch the ends together. Set the folded phyllo sheet on the baking pan, ruffles facing up. Repeat the process with seven or eight more sheets. Set them on the pan leaning against each other until the pan is full. Keep the remaining phyllo sheets covered. Bake for 10–12 minutes. Let the phyllo cool to room temperature. Leave the oven on.

- In a large bowl, whisk the eggs and the remaining sugar (not the cinnamon sugar). Whisk in the orange zest, vanilla, and orange liqueur. Whisk in the salt, baking powder, oil, and yogurt. Stir in the raisins. Shred the remaining phyllo sheets with your hands. Stir them into the yogurt mixture. Spread the mixture over the baked phyllo.

- Bake the pie on the middle rack for 35–40 minutes or until golden. Immediately ladle the reserved syrup over the portokalopita. Allow the phyllo pie to cool before serving.

# LOUKOUMADES (FRIED HONEY BALLS)

Serves 10

- 2 cups sugar
- 1 cup water
- 1 cup honey
- 1½ cups tepid water
- 1 tablespoon brown sugar
- ¼ cup vegetable oil
- 1 tablespoon active dry yeast
- 1½ cups all-purpose flour
- ½ cup cornstarch
- ⅛ teaspoon salt Vegetable oil for frying
- 1½ cups chopped walnuts
- ¼ cup ground cinnamon

**Directions**

- Bring the sugar and 1 cup water to a boil in a medium pot over medium-high heat. Then reduce the heat to medium and let it cook for 10 minutes. Add the honey, and allow the syrup to cool to room temperature and reserve it.
- In a large bowl, combine the tepid water, brown sugar, oil, and yeast. Set the mixture aside for 7–10 minutes to allow the yeast to activate. In another large bowl, combine the flour, cornstarch, and salt. Using a large wooden spoon or your hands, stir the flour mixture into the yeast to form wet dough. Cover the dough and let it rise in a warm place for 2 hours. The dough will be spongy.

- Set up a frying station: a glass of water, a teaspoon, and a deep frying pan. Heat 3 inches of oil in a deep frying pan over medium-high heat until the oil's temperature reaches 350°F. Adjust the heat to keep the temperature at 350°F while frying. Take a handful of dough in your palm, squeeze a small amount of dough onto the teaspoon (dunk the teaspoon in the water every so often), and drop the dough into the oil. Repeat with remaining dough. Fry for 3–4 minutes.

- Immediately after frying each batch, drop the loukoumades in the reserved syrup. Allow them to soak up the syrup for 3–4 minutes, and then place them on a rack over a baking pan to drain. Catch the excess syrup in the pan, and then add it back to the syrup bowl.

- Serve the loukoumades topped with the walnuts and cinnamon. Serve them warm or at room temperature.

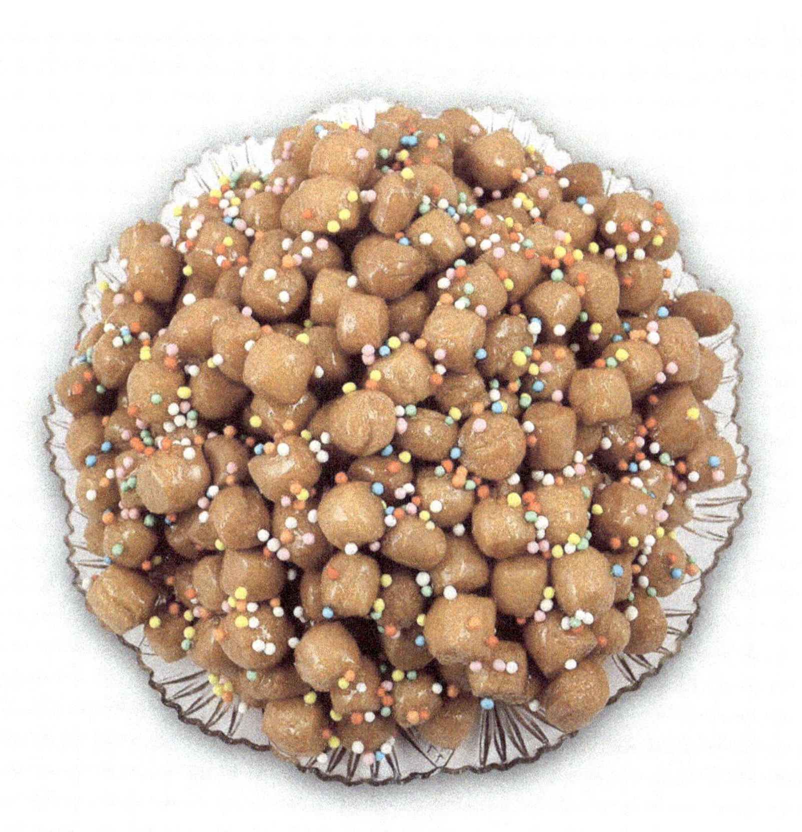

# MEDITERRANEAN BREAD

# LAHMACUN

Serves 8

- 1/2 large green bell pepper, stemmed, seeded, and chopped 1 medium red onion, peeled and chopped
- 2 cloves garlic, peeled and smashed
- 1 tablespoon red pepper paste
- 1 medium tomato, blanched, peeled, and chopped
- 1/2 pound ground lamb or beef
- 1 teaspoon salt
- 1/2 teaspoon pepper 1/2 teaspoon red pepper flakes
- 1 teaspoon ground allspice
- 1 teaspoon dried oregano
- 1/4 cup extra-virgin olive oil Pizza Dough
- 1/4 cup all-purpose flour

**Directions**

- Preheat the oven to 450°F. Set a pizza stone on the middle rack to preheat as well. If you don't have a pizza stone, use a large greased baking sheet.
- In a food processor, combine the peppers, onion, garlic, red pepper paste, and tomato. Pulse until the ingredients form a coarse paste. Add the ground lamb or beef, salt, pepper, red pepper flakes, allspice, oregano, and oil.
- Make sure the Pizza Dough has risen in a warm place for 11/2–2 hours. Punch down the dough and divide it into three pieces. Work with one piece of dough at a time. While one is baking, assemble the next one. Stretch and

flatten the dough into a long oval shape (about 10" × 4"). Transfer the dough to a well-floured pizza peel (paddle), which is a traditional Italian tool like a wide flat shovel, for moving a pizza so that the dough doesn't stick when you transfer it to the pizza stone (or baking sheet).

- Spread a third of the lamb filling over the top of the dough. Using your fingers, massage the filling into the dough, getting as near to the edges as possible. Carefully slide the lahmacun onto the pizza stone and bake it for 7–8 minutes or until the crust is browned. Repeat with the remaining dough and filling.
- Serve this dish hot or at room temperature.

# EASY HOMEMADE BREAD

Makes 3 loaves

- 2 tablespoons active dry yeast
- 1 teaspoon sugar
- 3½ cups tepid water
- 6¾ cups plus
- 2 tablespoons unbleached all-purpose flour, divided
- 1½ tablespoons salt
- 2 tablespoons coarse semolina flour

**Directions**

- In a large bowl, combine yeast, sugar, and water. Set aside for 7–10 minutes. Gradually stir in 6½ cups flour and salt until a dough starts to form. If the mixture seems a little dry, add up to ½ cup tepid water until the dough comes together. It should feel smooth and not too sticky. Cover the bowl with plastic wrap, leaving a small opening to allow the gases to escape. Let the dough rise a minimum of 2 hours or overnight.

- Sprinkle ¼ cup flour on a work surface. Divide dough into three pieces and work with one at a time. Stretch the dough outward and then fold under. Repeat this for 2–3 minutes. You should end up with a smooth, round ball (boule) of dough. Repeat with remaining dough.

- Sprinkle the semolina flour over a piece of parchment paper the same size as a pizza stone or baking sheet. Place the boules on the parchment, leaving room in between to allow the dough to rise. Sprinkle remaining flour over the boules. Let rise for 45 minutes. Use a sharp knife to cut three shallow slices into the top of each boule.

- Preheat the oven to 500°F. Set a pizza stone or large baking sheet on the middle rack to preheat. Add hot water to a broiler pan and place it on the top rack. Transfer the boules to the pizza stone or baking sheet and bake for 5 minutes. Reduce the temperature to 450°F and bake for 20 minutes or until the boules are golden.

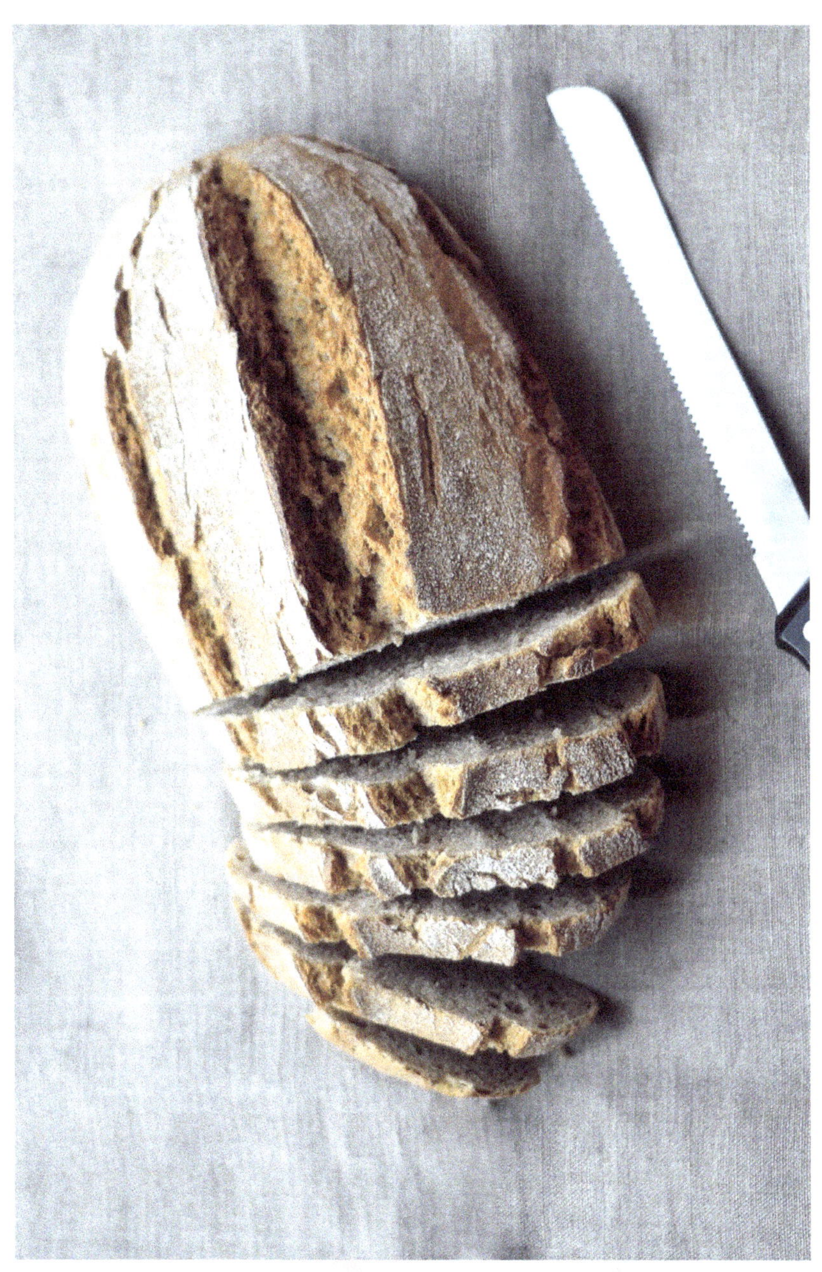

# MEDITERRANEAN RICE AND GRAINS

# Meyer Lemon Quinoa Skillet

## Ingredients

- 2 teaspoons olive oil
- 1⁄2 cup onion, chopped
- 1 teaspoon minced garlic
- 1 can (15.5 oz.) cannellini beans, drained and rinsed
- 1 can (14 oz.) quartered artichoke hearts, drained and roughly chopped
- 2 packages (10 oz.) Simple Truth Organic™ White Quinoa with Olive Oil & Sea Salt
- 1⁄4 cup water
- 2 Meyer lemons, zested and juiced
- 1⁄2 teaspoon salt
- 1⁄4 teaspoon ground black pepper
- 2 tablespoons flat leaf parsley, chopped
- 4 ounces crumbled feta cheese

## Directions

### Step 1

- In medium non-stick skillet over medium heat, heat oil. Cook onion and garlic 2 to 3 minutes, until translucent.

### Step 2

- Stir in beans, artichokes, quinoa and water. Cook 4 to 6 minutes until hot.

**Step 3**

- Stir in lemon juice, salt, pepper and parsley. Adjust seasoning to taste.

**Step 4**

- Serve topped with feta cheese and lemon zest.

# MEDITERRANEAN EGG AND RECIPIES

# Mediterranean-Breakfast-Burrito

**Ingredients**

- 6 tortillas whole 10 inch - I use sun-dried tomato
- 9 eggs whole
- 2 cups baby spinach washed and dried
- 3 tbsp black olives sliced
- 3 tbsp sun-dried tomatoes chopped
- ½ cup feta cheese I use light/low-fat feta
- ¾ cup refried beans canned
- Garnish: salsa (optional)

**Instructions**

- Spray medium frying pan with non- stick spray. Scramble eggs and toss for about 5 minutes, or until eggs are no longer liquid. Add spinach, black olives, sun-dried tomatoes and continue to stir/toss until no longer wet. Add feta cheese and cover until cheese is melted.
- Add 2 tbsp of refried beans to each tortilla. Top with egg mixture, dividing evenly between all burritos. Wrap as shown in video.
- Grill on panini press (this is what I use but you don't have to have one) or in frying pan until lightly browned.
- Serve hot with salsa and fruit (optional)
- If freezing: wait until cooled, then wrap as directed in video.
- If you are reheating: Heat in microwave (in parchment paper) for about 2 minutes. Serve hot.

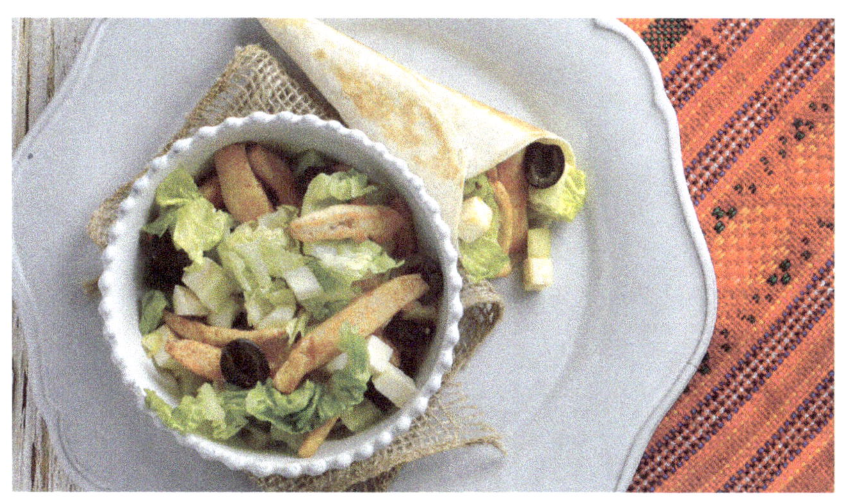

# MEDITERRANEAN BREAKFAST BAKE

# Easy Low Carb Bread Recipe (Almond Flour Bread)

**Ingredients**

- 2 cupWholesome Yum Blanched Almond Flour
- 1/4 cupPsyllium husk powder
- 1 tbspGluten-free baking powder
- 1/2 tspSea salt
- 4 large Eggs (beaten)
- 1/4 cupCoconut oil (measured solid, then melted)
- 1/2 cup Warm water

**Instructions**

1. Preheat the oven to 350 degrees F (177 degrees C). Line the bottom of a 9x5 in (23x13 cm) loaf pan with parchment paper.
2. In a large bowl, stir together the almond flour, psyllium husk powder, baking powder, and sea salt.
3. Stir in the eggs and melted coconut oil, then finally the warm water. Try to mix it well to create air bubbles.
4. Transfer the batter to the lined baking pan. Smooth/press the top evenly with your hands, forming a rounded top.
5. Bake for 55-70 minutes, until an inserted toothpick comes out clean and the top is very hard, like a bread crust. (Important: It will pass the toothpick test before it's completely done, so make sure the top is very crusty, too.) Cool completely before removing from the pan.

# Keto Low Carb Banana Bread Recipe With Almond Flour - Sugar Free

This low carb banana bread recipe with almond flour & coconut flour is perfectly moist & rich. No one will know it's keto banana bread! Naturally paleo, gluten-free, sugar-free, and healthy.

**Ingredients**

- 2 cupWholesome Yum Blanched Almond Flour
- 1/4 cupWholesome Yum Coconut Flour
- 1/2 cupWalnuts (chopped; plus more for topping if desired)
- 2 tspGluten-free baking powder
- 2 tspCinnamon
- 1/4 tspSea salt (optional)
- 6 tbspButter (softened; can use coconut oil for dairy-free, but flavor and texture will be different)
- 1/2 cupBesti Allulose *
- 1/2 tspXanthan gum
- 4 large Egg
- 1/4 cupUnsweetened almond milk
- 2 tspBanana extract

**Instructions**

1. Preheat the oven to 350 degrees F. Line a 9x5 in (23x13 cm) loaf pan with parchment paper, so that the paper hangs over two opposite sides (for easy removal later).
2. In a large bowl, mix together the almond flour, coconut flour, baking powder, cinnamon, and sea salt (if using).

3. In another large bowl, use a hand mixer to butter and sweetener until fluffy. Beat in the eggs (use the low setting to avoid splashing). Stir in the banana extract and almond milk.

4. Pour the dry ingredients into the wet. Beat on low setting until a dough/batter forms.

5. Stir in the chopped walnuts.

6. Transfer the batter into the lined loaf pan and press evenly to make a smooth top. If desired, sprinkle the top with additional chopped walnuts and press them lightly into the surface.

7. Bake for 50-60 minutes, until an inserted toothpick comes out clean.

8. Cool completely before removing from the pan and slicing. (The longer you let it sit before slicing, the better it will hold together. The next day is ideal if possible.)

# Keto Flaxseed Bread Recipe

This easy keto flaxseed bread recipe takes just 10 minutes to prep! It tastes like a nutty multi-grain bread, without any grains. Just 3g net carbs per slice!

**Ingredients**

- 3 cupsWholesome Yum Blanched Almond Flour
- 1 cupGolden flaxseed meal
- 1.5 tbspGluten-free baking powder
- 2 tbspBesti Monk Fruit Allulose Blend (optional, for better flavor)
- 1 tspSea salt
- 8 large Eggs (at room temperature)
- 1/2 cupButter (melted; use coconut oil for a dairy-free version)
- 1 cup Warm water
- 1/2 cupFlax seeds (optional, plus more for sprinkling on top if desired)

**Instructions**

1. Preheat the oven to 350 degrees F (177 degrees C). Line the bottom of a 9x5 in (23x13 cm) loaf pan with parchment paper.
2. In a large bowl, stir together the almond flour, flaxseed meal, baking powder, Besti, and sea salt.
3. Stir in the eggs and melted butter, then finally the warm water. Try to mix it well to create air bubbles. Stir in the flax seeds.

4.  Transfer the batter to the lined baking pan. Smooth the top evenly, forming a rounded top. Sprinkle more flax seeds over top if desired.

5.  Bake for 45-50 minutes, until an inserted toothpick comes out clean and the top is crusty and brown. (Important: It will pass the toothpick test before it's completely done, so make sure the top is very crusty, too.) Cool completely before removing from the pan.

6.

# Almond Flour Keto Blueberry Bread Recipe

Keto lemon blueberry bread is like a low carb blueberry muffin loaf! With just 10 minutes prep in ONE BOWL, almond flour blueberry bread tastes just like the coffee shop, right at home.

**Ingredients**

- 2 1/2 cupsWholesome Yum Blanched Almond Flour
- 1/2 cupBesti Monk Fruit Allulose Blend
- 1/2 tbspGluten-free baking powder
- 1/2 tspXanthan gum (optional, but recommended for structure)
- 1/4 tspSea salt
- 1/3 cupUnsweetened almond milk
- 1/3 cupButter (melted; use coconut oil for dairy-free option)
- 3 large Eggs (at room temperature)
- 1/2 tspVanilla extract
- 1 medium Lemon (juiced and zested; use 1 tbsp zest and 1 tbsp juice)
- 3/4 cup Blueberries
- 1/3 cupBesti Powdered Monk Fruit Allulose Blend

**Instructions**

1. Preheat the oven to 350 degrees F (176 degrees C). Line a 8x4 loaf pan with parchment paper, with the paper hanging over at least the two long sides.

2.  In a large bowl, stir together the dry ingredients - almond flour, sweetener, baking powder, xanthan gum (if using), and sea salt.

3.  Stir in the almond milk, melted butter, eggs, and vanilla, until smooth. Stir in the lemon zest (no juice). Fold in the blueberries.

4.  Transfer the batter into the lined loaf pan. Press evenly to make a smooth top.

5.  Bake for 40 minutes. Tent the top with foil, then continue baking for 10-15 minutes, until an inserted toothpick comes out clean. Let the bread cool completely before moving out of the pan.

In a small bowl, make the glaze by whisking together 1 tablespoon lemon juice (15 ml) and powdered sweetener. If glaze is too runny, add more sweetener a bit at a time until

# MEDITERRANEAN APPETIZERS

# Creamy Cucumbers

Total time: 15 minutes

Prep time: 15 minutes

Cook time: 0 minutes

Yield: 4 servings

**Ingredients**

- 2 English cucumbers, thinly sliced

- 1 ½ cups low-fat Greek yogurt

- 2 tbsp. lemon juice, fresh

- 1 ½ tsp. mustard seeds

- Coarse salt and ground pepper, to taste   Small bunch dill

**Directions**

Combine all the ingredients in a bowl until well combined.

# Roasted Veggie Hummus

Total time: 1 hour

Prep time: 20 minutes

Cook time: 40 minutes

Yields: 20 servings

**Ingredients**

- 1 bulb garlic
- ¾ cup olive oil, divided
- 1 egg plant, halved
- 1 red bell pepper, halved
- ⅓ cup lemon juice, freshly squeezed
- 2 cans chickpeas, drained
- ¼ cup sesame tahini paste
- ⅓ tsp. smoked paprika
- ½ tsp. salt

**Direction**

- Heat your oven to 450°F and line a baking pan with foil.
- Cut the very top of the garlic bulb off and drizzle with 1 teaspoon of olive oil.
- Next wrap it up in foil.
- On a separate pan, place the eggplant and bell pepper, drizzle with 2 tablespoons of olive oil, and toss so it coats evenly.

- Place the wrapped garlic into the pan containing the vegetables.
- Roast for 30 minutes without covering and cool for 10 minutes.
- Remove the peels from eggplant and bell pepper and chop the vegetables into small pieces.
- Place the chickpeas in a food processor with a metal blade and process until smooth.
- Next, squeeze the pulp from the garlic into the processor; add all the other ingredients including the roasted vegetables and process until well blended.  Serve into small serving bowls and serve immediately and refrigerate the remainder.